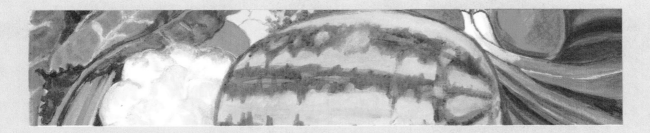

"The Doctors in Mili's Suitcase is an important story about the power of plant-based foods. Katherine Orr does a wonderful job of describing diabetes and how it can be tackled with food. Rates of diabetes are increasing every day, and children younger and younger are being diagnosed with a disease easily prevented by eating a low-fat plant-based diet. Our studies at the Physicians Committee for Responsible Medicine have shown that a vegan diet helps to reverse type 2 diabetes. Let Mili be your role model for taking control of your health and transforming your life with a plant-based diet."

–*Neal Barnard, M.D.*
  President, Physicians Committee for Responsible Medicine

Important: A person who is on medication should be under medical supervision when changing diet because blood sugar levels can normalize quickly as the person becomes healthier.
The information in this book is for educational purposes only. It is not intended to be a substitute for professional medical advice.

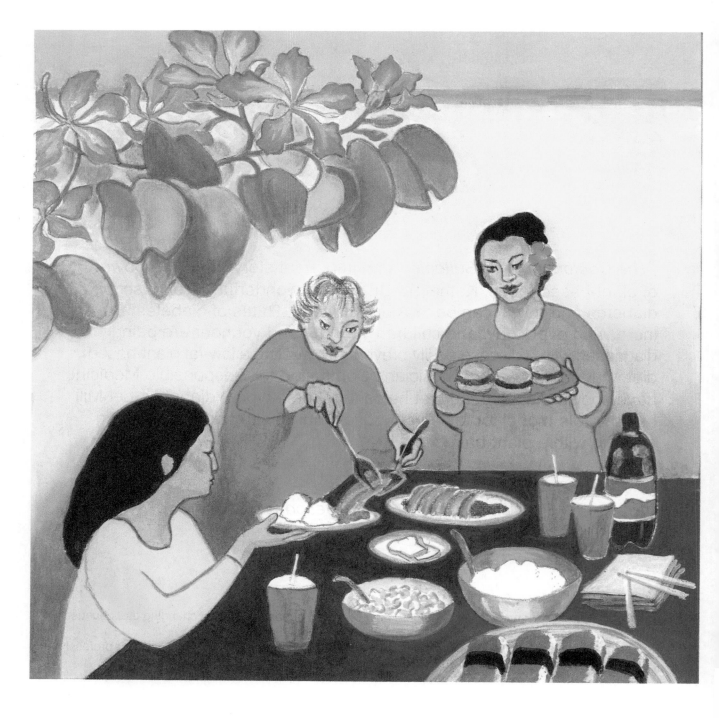

THE DOCTORS IN MILI'S SUITCASE

How I Cured My Diabetes With Food

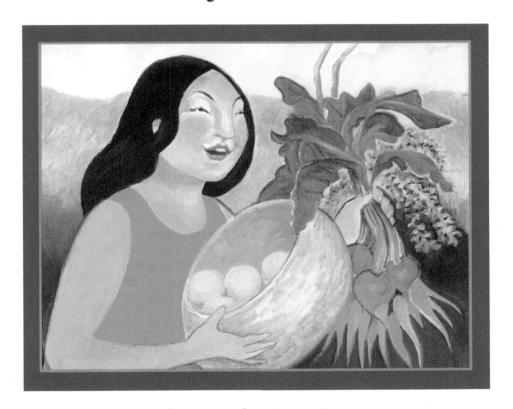

by Katherine Orr

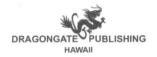

DRAGONGATE PUBLISHING
HAWAII

ISBN: 978-0-9765178-4-9

DragonGate Publising
44-119 Bayview Haven Place
Kaneohe, HI 96744
Published and printed in the United States of America   Second edition

www.katherineshelleyorr.com

Orr, Katherine Shelley
THE DOCTORS IN MILI'S SUITCASE, How I Cured My Diabetes With Food / written and illustrated by Katherine Orr

ISBN: 978-0-9765178-4-9 (standard paperback)
ISBN: 978-0-9765178-3-2 (premium paperback)

Summary: An eleven-year-old girl learns about food's power to cause, prevent, and reverse disease. She heals herself from type-2 diabetes by changing the foods she eats.

to Mili

a 'read aloud' book for family sharing and learning

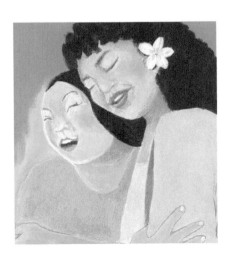

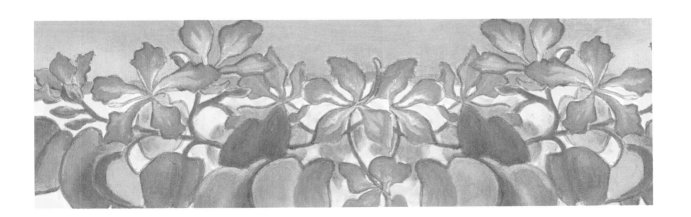

"Food can say 'I love you' in a million different ways." That's what Grandma Tutu always said. *Tutu* means grandparent in Hawaiian. Tutu's favorite thing was sharing loving gifts of food. "When we celebrate, food can say, 'Well done!'" she explained. "When someone's hurting, food can say, 'I hope you're feeling better.'"

We all knew food was a gift of love... but a gift of health? Well, I never thought about it. At least not until the year I turned eleven. That was the year I got diabetes.

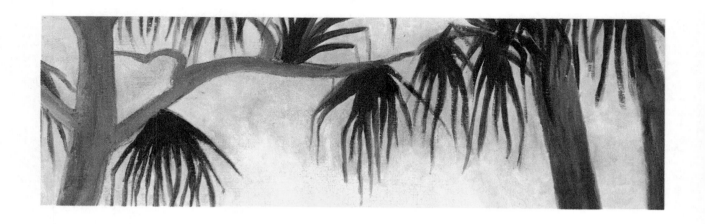

Mom said, "Diabetes is in our genes. Tutu has it, and your Uncle Kim. But you, my baby, are still so young." She hugged me and her eyes were sad. "Hana, I'll help you learn to live with diabetes."

And for a while she did just that – until Mom's sister, Mili, came to visit. She stayed for the summer and everything changed. Professor Mili and the doctors in her suitcase showed me how to live *without* diabetes!

Here's the way it happened.

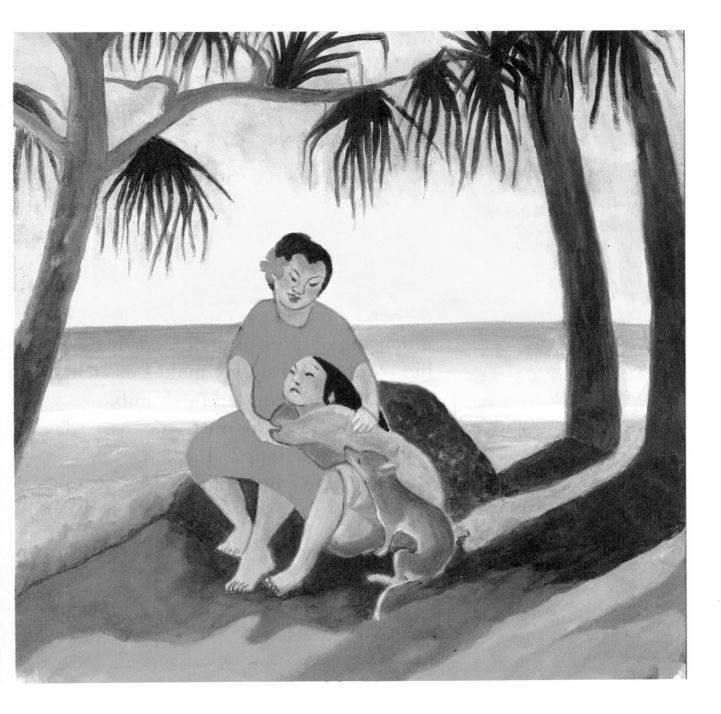

Insulin is like a key that unlocks the cell door so sugar can go inside the cell, where it's burned for energy or stored as fat. In type 1 diabetes, the body doesn't make enough insulin, so there's no key to unlock the cell door. In type 2 diabetes—the kind Hana has—the body makes insulin. The key is there, but the door lock is jammed so the key doesn't work well.

Type 2 diabetes used to be called 'adult onset' diabetes because it occurred only in adults. Now so many children have the disease that many experts don't use that name anymore.

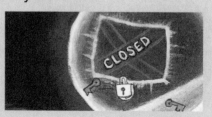

When the doctor told me the diagnosis, he explained diabetes like this:

After we eat, our blood sugar rises. Then insulin moves the sugar from our blood into our cells. When we have diabetes, insulin isn't doing its job. Too much sugar stays in the blood. It causes big trouble and slowly makes us sick.

Then he dropped the bomb...
"You'll need to take medicine every day."
"For how long?" I asked.
"For life," he replied.

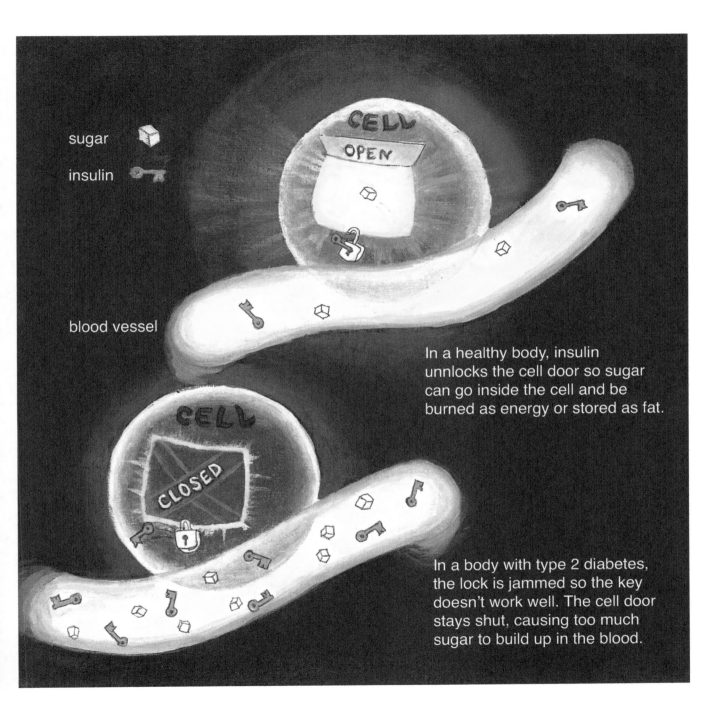

sugar

insulin

blood vessel

In a healthy body, insulin unnlocks the cell door so sugar can go inside the cell and be burned as energy or stored as fat.

In a body with type 2 diabetes, the lock is jammed so the key doesn't work well. The cell door stays shut, causing too much sugar to build up in the blood.

When Hana was diagnosed with diabetes, her doctor said the disease was incurable. He told Hana diabetes could be managed with the help of medicines, exercise, and a special diet. He said most diabetes gets slowly worse. After a while, pills might not be sufficient to keep the blood sugar normal. Other medicines might also be needed to protect the heart, kidneys, and other organs from damage.

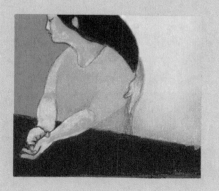

I was scared this meant sticking a needle in my skin. That's what Uncle Kim and Tutu did. But the doctor gave me pills instead. He said, "Eat right, lose weight, exercise, and get sound sleep. These things will help you manage your disease."

He gave Mom and me a booklet called *Diabetes Diet*. It was full of instructions about counting carbs and calories, and it had lots of numbers that I didn't understand. But one thing I did know: if I didn't control my blood sugar, I could wind up blind, or paralyzed from a stroke like my Uncle Kim. Or with leg and kidney problems like Tutu had.

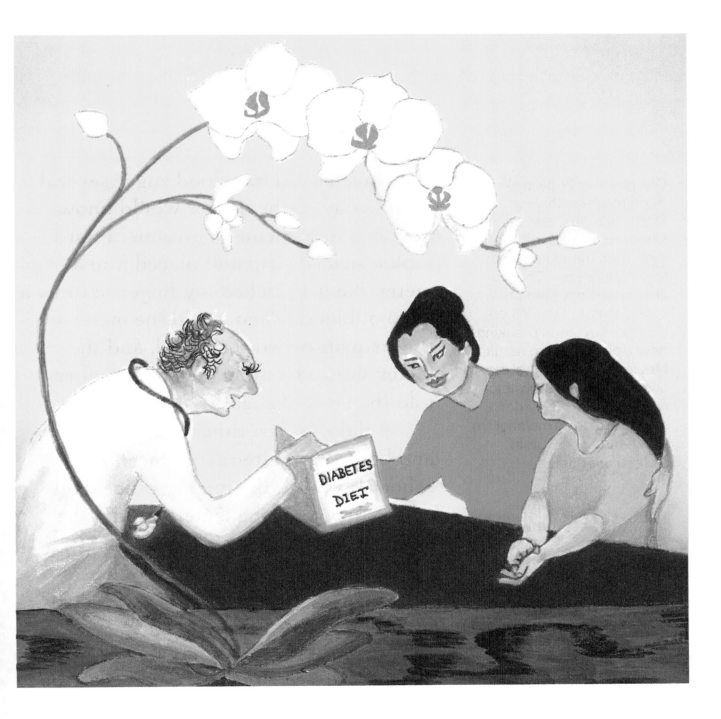

Our physical body is like a living machine that runs on food, water, air, and attitude. Chemical processes in our cells burn the food we eat to create energy. These chemical processes are called *metabolism*. When metabolism starts breaking down, diabetes can result. Medicines that control blood sugar treat only a symptom, not the cause. They don't repair the body's metabolism, which may continue to worsen over time.

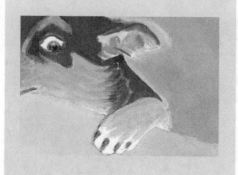

I measured my blood sugar several times a day so the doctor would know how much medicine to give me. First I took a special strip and placed it in a meter. Next I pricked my finger to draw a drop of blood. Then I held the meter so the strip absorbed the blood, and the meter showed a number. That number told the level of sugar in my blood.

I did this first thing every morning, and before and after every meal. At school I went to the nurses' office daily, where they kept the meter and did the blood test for me.

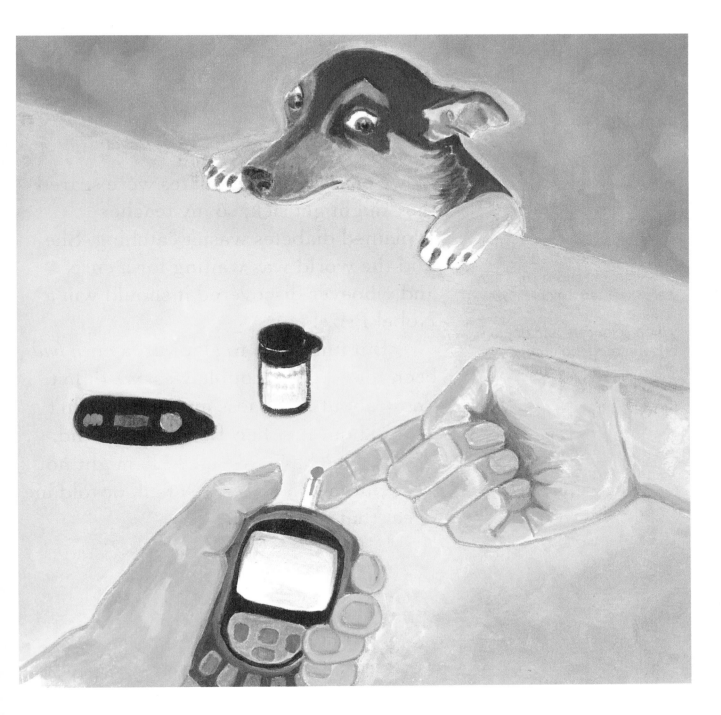

In the early 1920s, two scientists discovered insulin and used it to manage the symptoms of diabetes. Their work was celebrated as a breakthrough, and in 1923 they were awarded a Nobel Prize.

When scientists and doctors encountered the *cure* for diabetes—a cure that repaired and strengthened the metabolism—the news was not widely reported or celebrated.

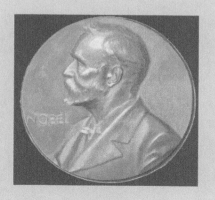

Some of my classmates were scared they might get sick, so my teacher explained diabetes wasn't catching. She said the world was waiting for a cure, and whoever discovered it should win a Nobel Prize.

But unknown to all of us, a cure *had* been found. The trouble was, we didn't know about it. I guess my doctor didn't know about it either. Because if he did, wouldn't he have told me? He might not have put me on medicine at all, or told me to eat that diabetes diet.

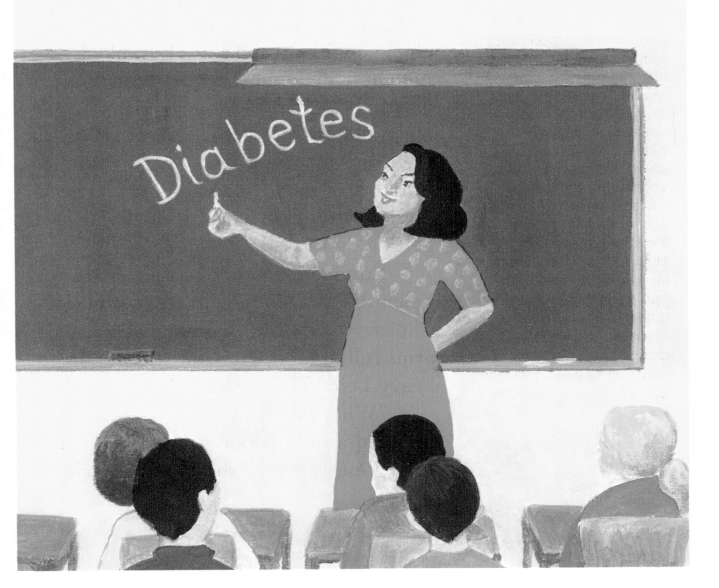

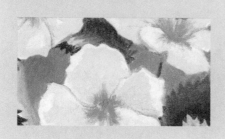

On the diabetes diet I was always watching what I ate. I ate steamed white chicken without the skin. I drank skim milk and ate low-fat yogurt. For snacks I drank diet soda, and my cookies were always sugar free. I tried to eat small, but the less I ate, the more I was always thinking of food. I was gaining weight, not losing it. And worst of all, I was getting depressed.

Summer vacation was just starting when Aunty Mili flew over from Hilo. She arrived on our doorstep with her arms full of food. Her suitcase was so heavy I could barely lift it.

"What's *in* this thing?" I asked as I dragged it in the door.

"Open and see!" she said with a grin.

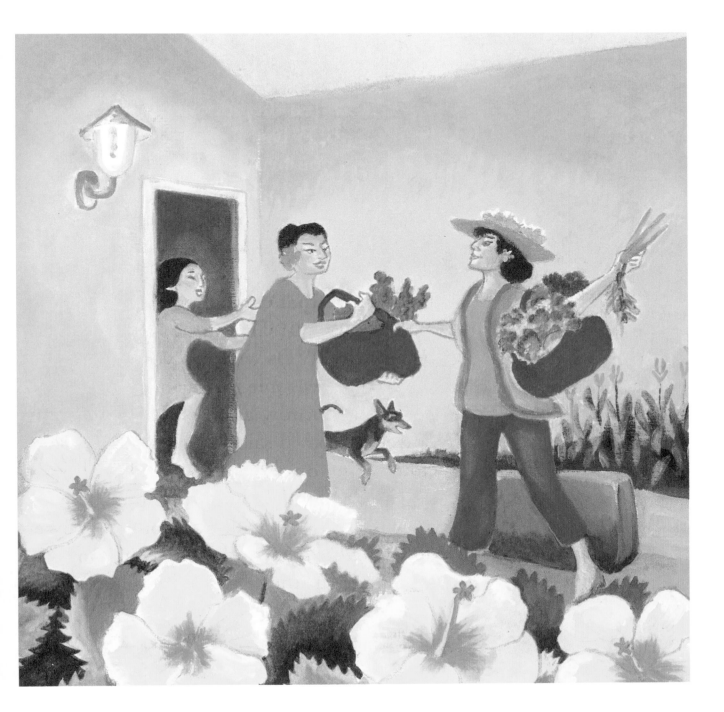

.

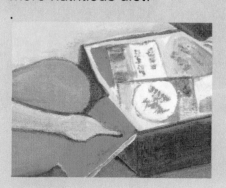

As I lifted the lid, out spilled colorful books and DVDs.

"Did you bring stories and movies to make us laugh?" I asked.

Aunty Mili shook her head. "These books and DVDs are something much more special. They hold knowledge, Hana. Knowledge that can change your life and make you well! The authors of these books and DVDs will help you understand about the awesome power of food!"

"Oh, I know all about the awesome power of food," I said, gazing at the vanilla cake sitting on the counter. It was Mom's special gift to welcome Mili home.

"Ho! You're talking about the power of food *addiction*," said Mili. "But I'm talking about the power of whole food, plant-based *nutrition*."

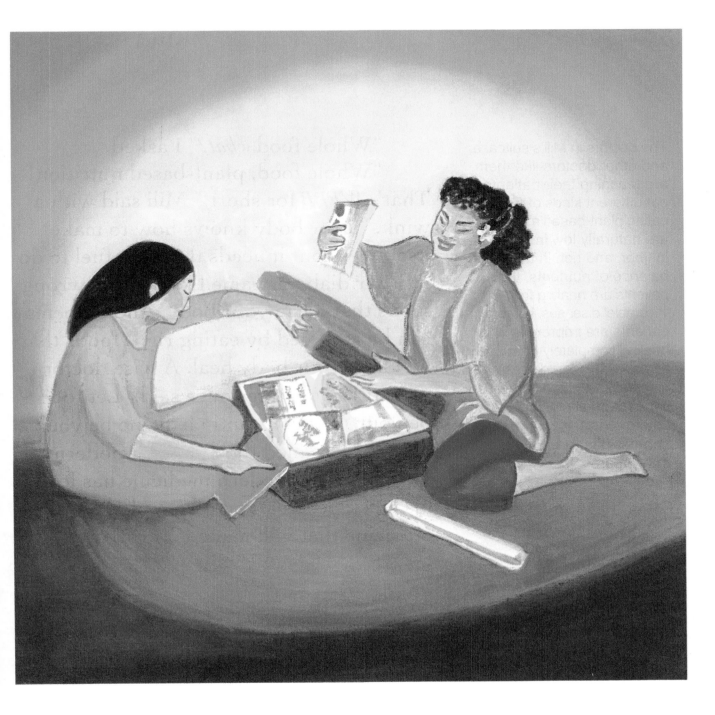

The doctors in Mili's suitcase, and other doctors like them, are teaching their patients to eat different kinds of food. By eating plant-based meals that are naturally low in fat, high in fiber, and rich in the right balance of nutrients, their patients are healing from 'incurable' diseases. In fact, patients are improving and healing completely from such ailments as heart disease, diabetes, high blood pressure, cancers, multiple sclerosis, osteoporosis, gallstones, depression, arthritis... and many more.

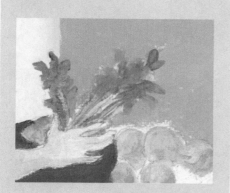

"Whole food *what?*" I asked.

"Whole food, plant-based nutrition! That's *WFPB* for short," Mili said with a wink. "Your body knows how to make itself well, but it needs the right fuel to do it. Your diabetes came from eating wrong foods that harm your body. And diabetes can be reversed by eating right foods that will help your body heal. A wise doctor named Hippocrates once said, 'Let food be your medicine, and medicine be your food.' He's called the father of modern medicine, but modern medicine has lost his message. Real food from plants *is* the medicine that will make you well."

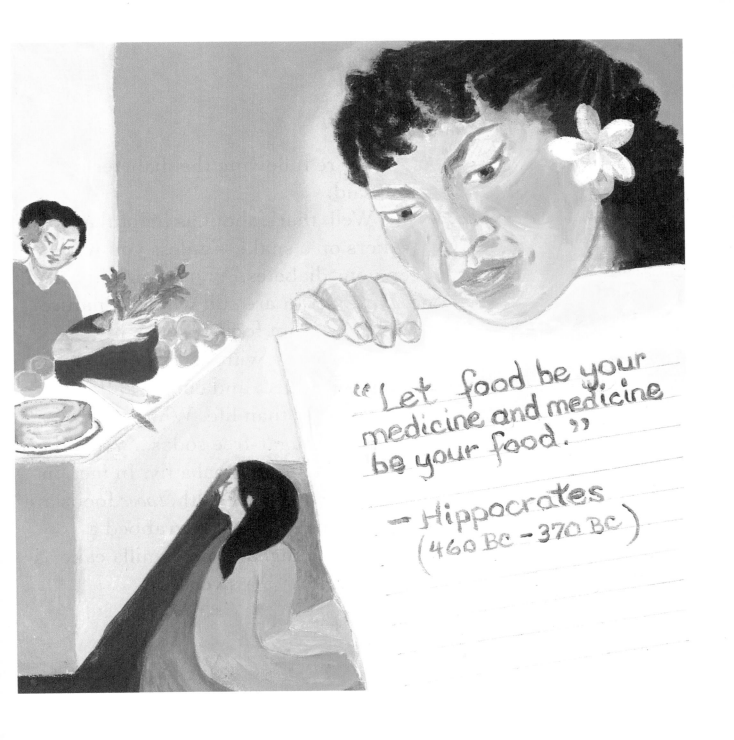

What makes plants such powerful medicine? Here's a clue: scientists have identified more than one hundred thousand (*yes! one hundred thousand!*) protective nutrients found *only* in plants. These healing nutrients work together like the notes in a symphony: they create health effects that are greater than the sum of their parts. Many processed plant foods have been stripped of important nutrients and contain added harmful ingredients. In highly processed foods, the living symphony once found within the plant has been reduced to a lifeless jumble of notes.

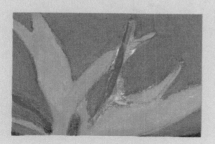

"We're following the diabetes diet..." Mom said.

"Well, that's about as helpful as sneakers on a snake – unless you want to keep your diabetes," chuckled Mili. "You need foods that are still whole as nature made them – not food-like inventions made in a factory, with key parts removed, extra parts added, and chemical flavors that are larger than life. White flour cookies and sugar-free sodas... Why, those foods couldn't even heal a fly. In fact, in the fight for Hana's health, *those* foods are on the wrong side!" Mili grabbed a parsnip and lunged at the vanilla cake as if stabbing it with a sword.

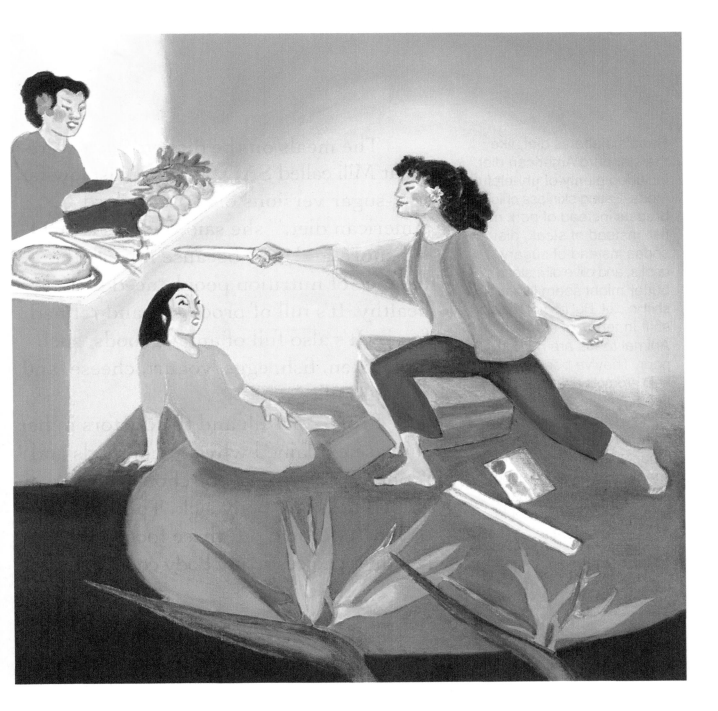

Hana's diabetes diet, like the standard American diet, included plenty of unhelpful foods. Eating skinless chicken breasts instead of pork ribs, fish instead of steak, diet sodas instead of sugary drinks, and olive oil instead of butter might seem like a big shift in diet. But it's not a major shift in terms of nutrition. Animal foods are nutrient-poor. They've been shown to help promote diabetes, cancer, heart disease, and more. Hana was eating animal foods daily, as well as processed foods, including oils. And she was not eating enough nutrient-rich whole foods from plants. A diet like this could not reverse her disease.

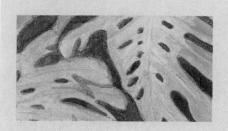

The meals on the diabetes diet were what Mili called SAD. "They're just low-fat, low-sugar versions of the 'standard American diet,'" she said. "That's S-A-D for short, and *SAD* because it lacks the balance of nutrition people need to stay healthy. It's full of processed and refined foods. It's also full of animal foods, such as chicken, fish, eggs, yogurt, cheese, and low-fat milk."

Professor Mili and the doctors in her suitcase explained why animal foods and refined foods were poor choices that helped keep my body sick. They showed us how to crowd out these foods with healthier choices so my body could get well.

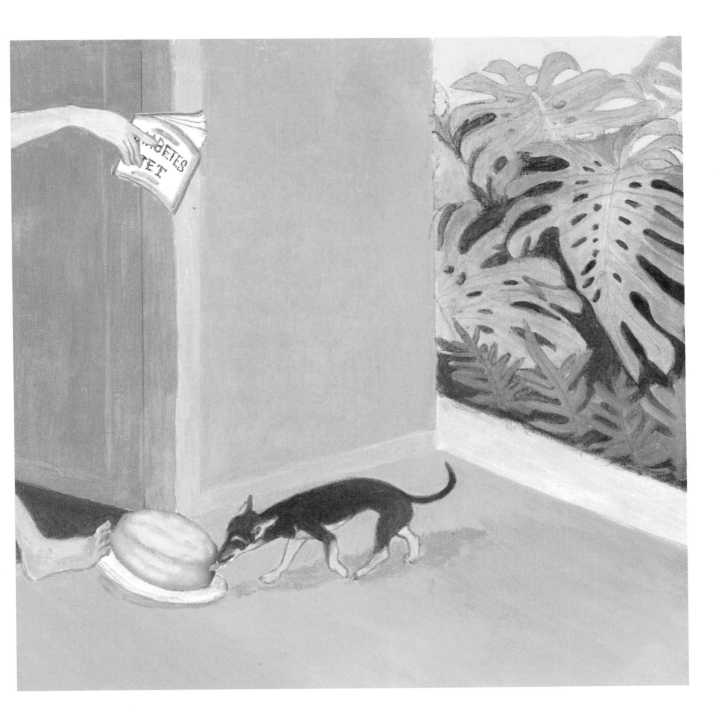

Throughout history, the diets of all large, successful, long-lasting civilizations have always centered on plants. Legumes, whole grains, roots, tubers, and starchy vegetables have been the main source of calories (energy) in the human diet. Native Americans ate corn and beans. Native Hawaiians ate taro and sweet potatoes. Ancient Romans ate barley and wheat, and ancient Asians ate whole-grain rice and millet.

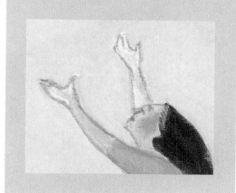

Mili did a quick spin and tossed me an orange. "The food you eat becomes your body. If you want a junk body, eat junk food. If you want a body that's a clean and lean self-healing machine, then feed it with fuel that's designed for the job. When you learn which types of foods to eat, you can eat all you want and still lose weight. You won't have to count carbs or calories. Your cravings for junk food will disappear. Your taste buds will change, and the food will taste scrumptious. Mark my words!"

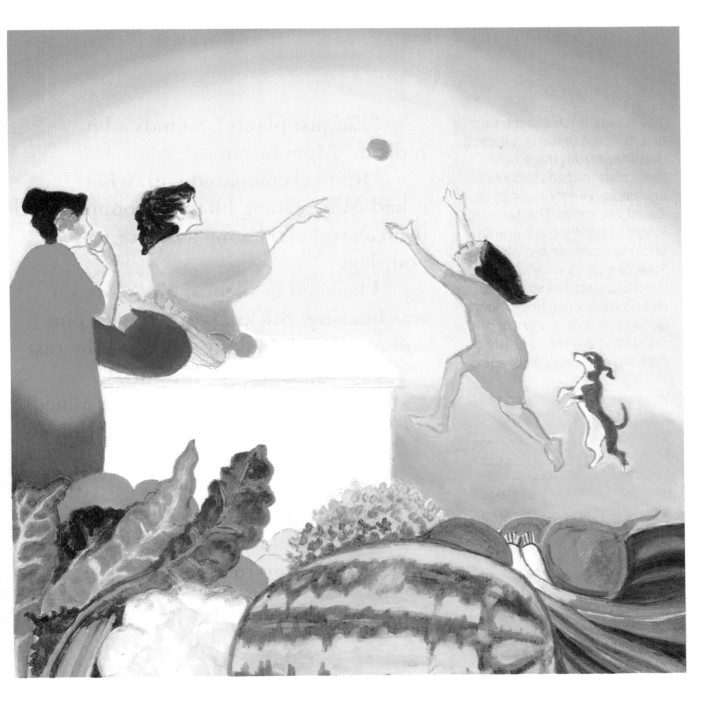

The American diet of the past one hundred years is a radical departure from the whole food, plant-based diets of our ancestors. But for most of us, it's all we know. The familiar foods eaten by our parents and grandparents are what we think of as a 'normal' diet. The familiar diseases this harmful diet promotes (including heart disease, diabetes, cancer and dementia) we mistakenly think are a normal part of aging.

When a baby is born it prefers the flavors of foods its mother ate while pregnant. So the best time for a mother to start helping her child love to eat healthy food begins with what *she* eats while she is pregnant.

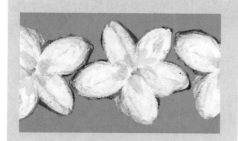

"Eat just plants? Sounds a bit radical," Mom began.

"Radical compared with what?" asked Mili. "Going blind? Dropping dead from a stroke? Having a doctor cut off your legs?"

I listened in silence, but my brain was buzzing. Sticking myself with pins and needles and taking medicine the rest of my life – wasn't *that* radical?

I felt confused, but also determined. I gave Aunty Mili a giant hug. "If doing this can make me well, then I want to do it with all my heart!"

That night I almost couldn't sleep knowing the cure for diabetes was sitting right in my living room.

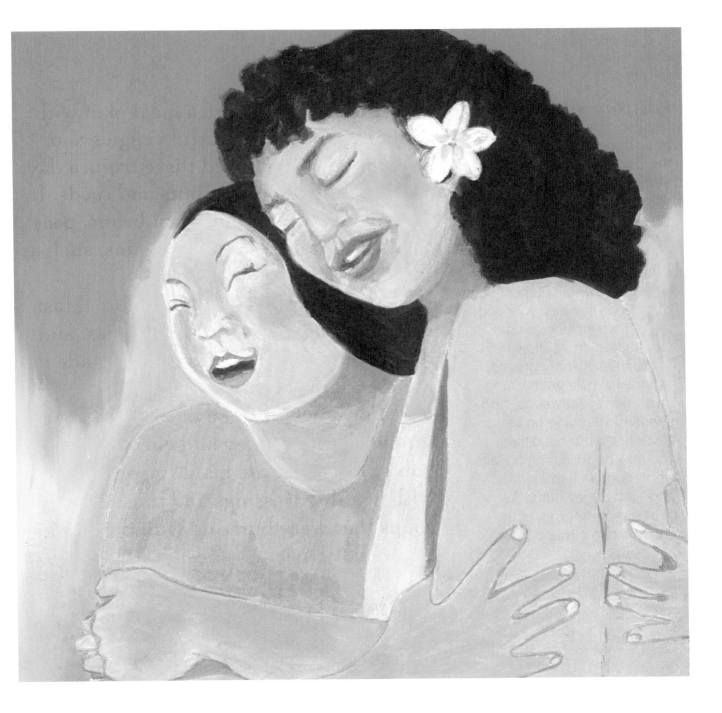

Each doctor in Mili's suitcase had his or her own recipes and suggestions. But overall, the doctors shared a single strong message: Fill up on whole plant foods—they move you towards health. Let them crowd out animal foods and refined foods, which move you towards disease. What are the high-fiber, low-fat, nutrient-rich plant foods that help your body heal? They include colorful vegetables, fruits, flowers, roots, tubers, leafy greens, legumes, whole grains, fungi, mushrooms, seaweeds, and seeds. Depending on the severity of your condition, you may need to omit certain whole foods such as nuts and high-sugar fruits. As your health returns, your choices can expand.

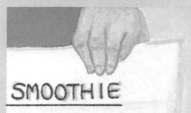

SMOOTHIE

Mom and I chose a meal plan with unlimited loads of colorful veggies and leafy greens. It allowed three fruits a day, plus a small amount of nuts and seeds. It had lots of different kinds of beans, peas, and lentils, and also whole grains, such as oats and rice.

Instead of eating eggs for breakfast, we ate oatmeal topped with berries, and drank velvety green smoothies I made in the blender.

For lunch, instead of a skimpy sandwich with turkey and cheese plus a gob of mayo, we ate giant crispy salads with healthy dressings and thick, chunky soups that were bursting with flavor.

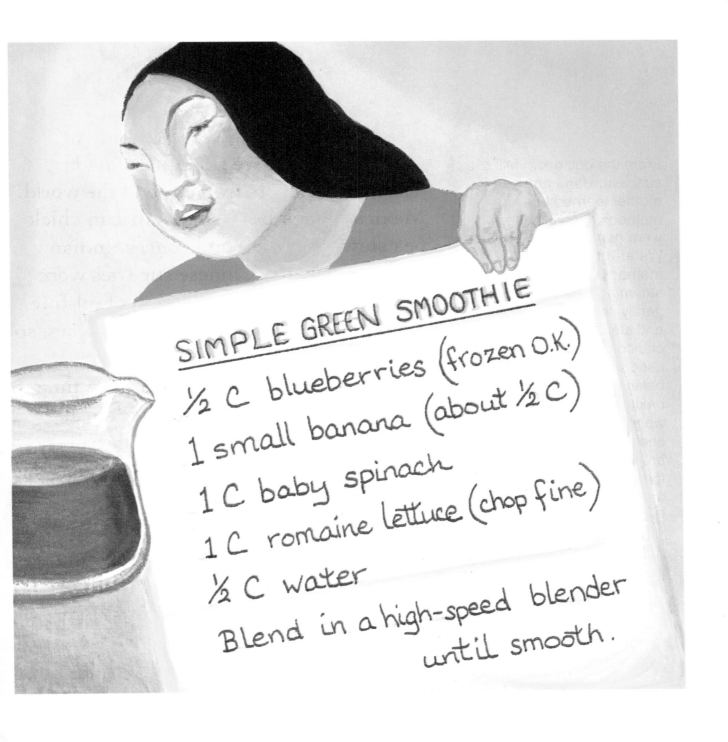

From the doctors in Mili's suitcase, Hana and her mother learned that some methods of cooking foods were healthier than others. Water-based cooking methods—such as lightly steaming vegetables and gently simmering soups and stews—were healthier choices than methods that used hot, dry heat, such as baking and toasting. Gentle baking without browning and warm-air drying were healthier choices than hot grilling and broiling, which scorch the food. Steam frying was a healthy replacement for frying with oil.

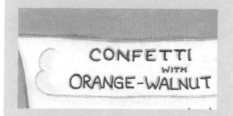

CONFETTI
WITH
ORANGE-WALNUT

For dinner, we sometimes made dishes with flavors from around the world. Mexican black bean soup, African chick pea stew, Thai vegetable curry, Indian split-pea dal, and Chinese stir-fries were part of our growing collection of oil-free recipes. We made enough for leftovers, so we didn't need to cook every day.

On days when we didn't have time to cook, we ate leftovers or served meals that were fast and easy, such as taro or pumpkin with a pile of steamed greens, or confetti salad and a side of beans. By keeping frozen vegetables, spices, beans, grains, and fruits on hand we could make interesting, healthy meals in minutes.

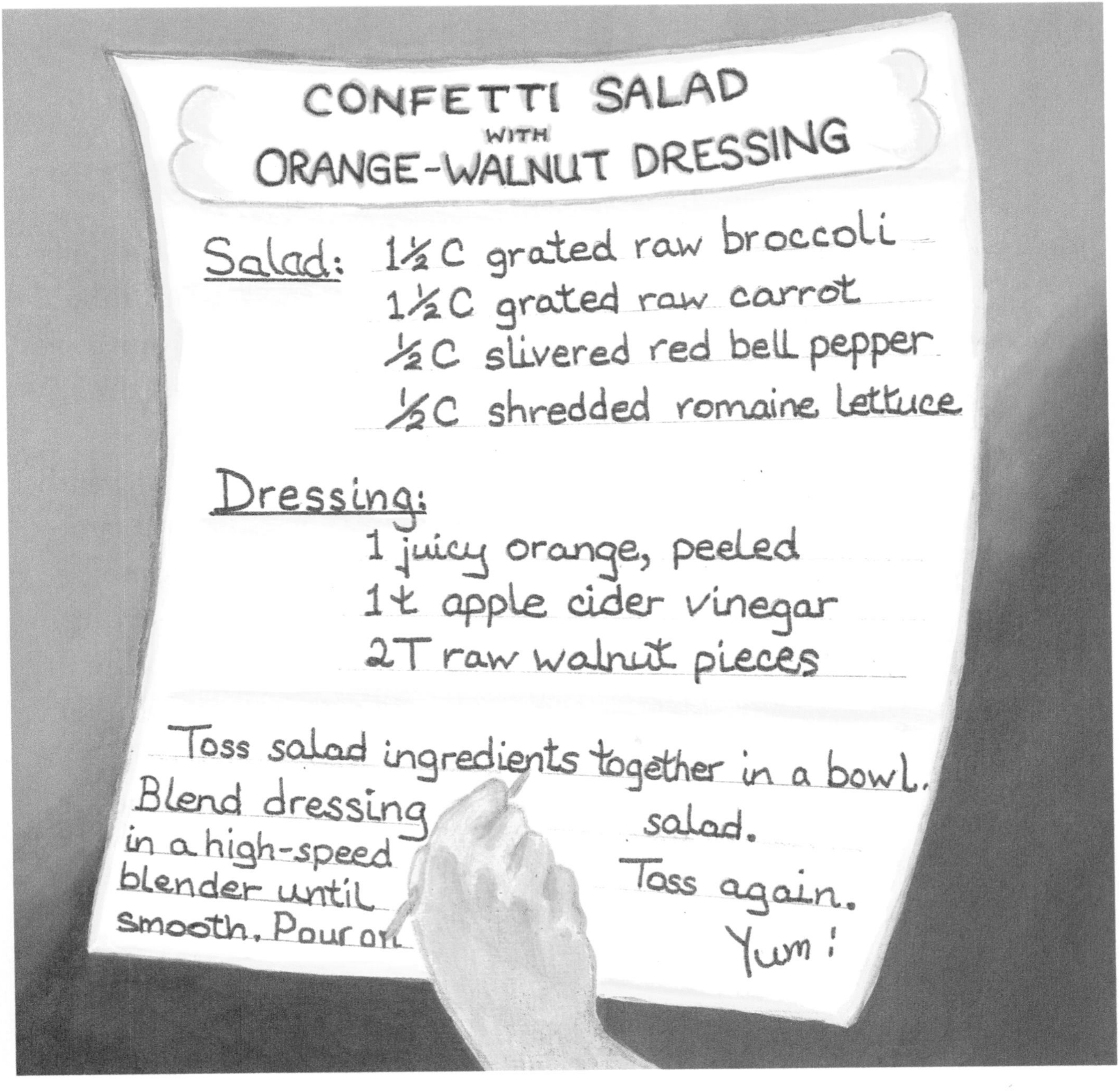

CONFETTI SALAD
WITH
ORANGE-WALNUT DRESSING

Salad:
- 1½ C grated raw broccoli
- 1½ C grated raw carrot
- ½ C slivered red bell pepper
- ½ C shredded romaine lettuce

Dressing:
- 1 juicy orange, peeled
- 1 t apple cider vinegar
- 2 T raw walnut pieces

Toss salad ingredients together in a bowl.
Blend dressing in a high-speed blender until smooth. Pour on salad.
Toss again.
Yum!

It may seem easier just to take a pill, but a lifetime of buying medicine and supplies is expensive and preventable. And controlling blood sugar with medicine is not the same as becoming healthy. When you continue to eat the same diet that caused your diabetes, the disease will continue to progress. Damage will spread throughout the body. Taking medicine without changing the source of the problem is like squirting water on flames while continuing to pour gasoline on the fire.

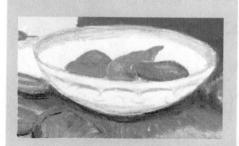

We started calling this Our Great Food Adventure. We laughed and talked story as we washed and chopped our food.

"All this chopping sure takes time," I said.

Aunty Mili quickly nabbed me with her eyes. "Hana, which takes more time *and* more money: making wholesome meals that keep you healthy and strong, or juggling medicines and visits to the doctor? And which makes for a happier life?"

I smiled and nodded. Some questions don't need answers.

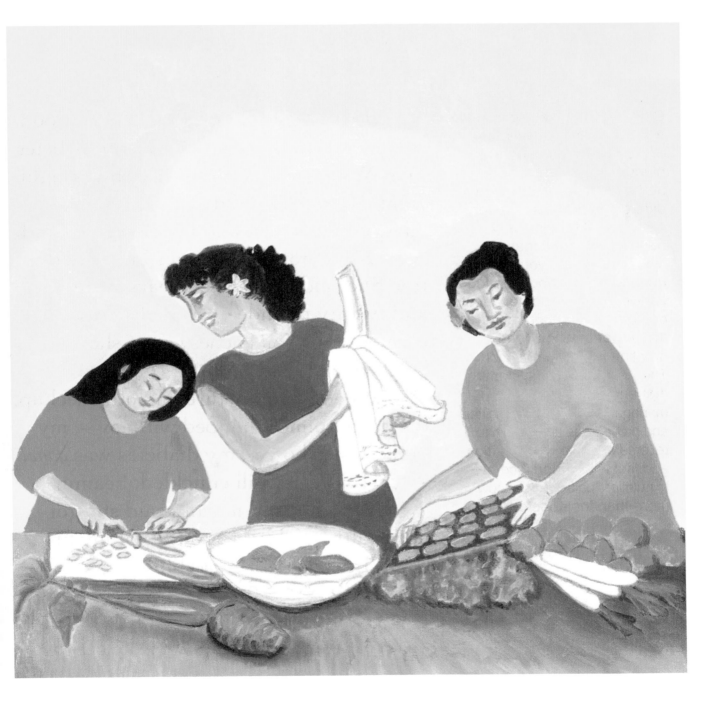

Compared with taking medicines for life, eating a diet of whole foods from plants is powerful, simple, and safe. It doesn't require a different food to target every symptom. It brings many benefits without negative side effects, and you don't need to worry about one food conflicting with another. Most doctors aren't taught about the power of whole food nutrition in medical school. They work within a system that encourages them to manage disease with medicines and procedures rather than to reverse disease with nutrition and lifestyle. When it comes to nutrition, patients can know more than their doctors do.

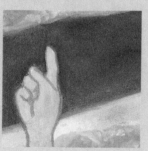

Just one week into Our Great Food Adventure, the doctor took me off diabetes pills. With each passing week, my weight went down. My mind got clearer, my allergies vanished, and my energy soared.

Mom noticed changes in her body, too. She said she felt ten years younger and twenty pounds lighter. "Energy up, pounds down, joint aches gone," she laughed.

When I had my three-month checkup, the doctor almost jumped with joy – my blood tests showed my diabetes was *gone!*

"Told ya," Mili chuckled, beaming.

Mom hugged me and said she got her healthy girl back. And I got my life back. In fact, I got a *new* life!

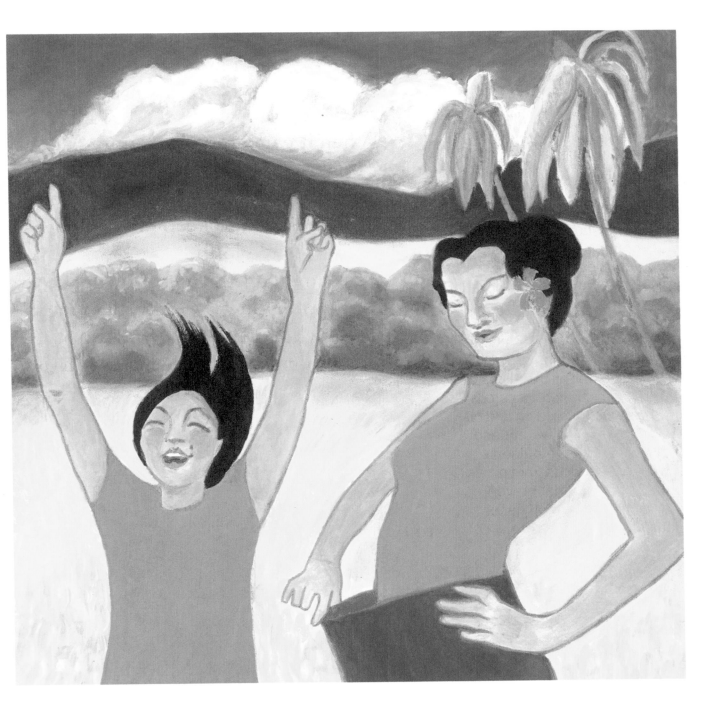

Nobody has perfect genes. Despite this, most of us live normal lives. Genes are not as poweful as scientists once thought. They're like sets of instructions that can't act on their own. Signals from outside the genes turn them on and off and tell them what to do. This field of study is called *epigenetics*. Epigeneticists know that our lifestyles and diets affect our genes, as well as the genes of our unborn children. Hundreds of genes are turned on and off with every meal we eat and digest. Protective nutrients within whole foods from plants turn on genes that prevent disease and turn off genes that promote disease.

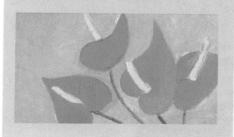

When it came time for Aunty Mili to leave, I had no words to thank her for all that she'd done. I just held her tight for a long time and tried to keep my wet cheeks off her silk travel blouse.

As Mom hugged Aunty Mili goodbye, she said, "All my life I've been blaming our genes, when our *food* is what turns those genes on and off! We all have a few bad genes of some kind, but bad genes can't hurt us when they're turned off. I sure wish I'd known this a long time ago. It's less about the *genes* that run in our family than the *eating styles* we pass on to our kids."

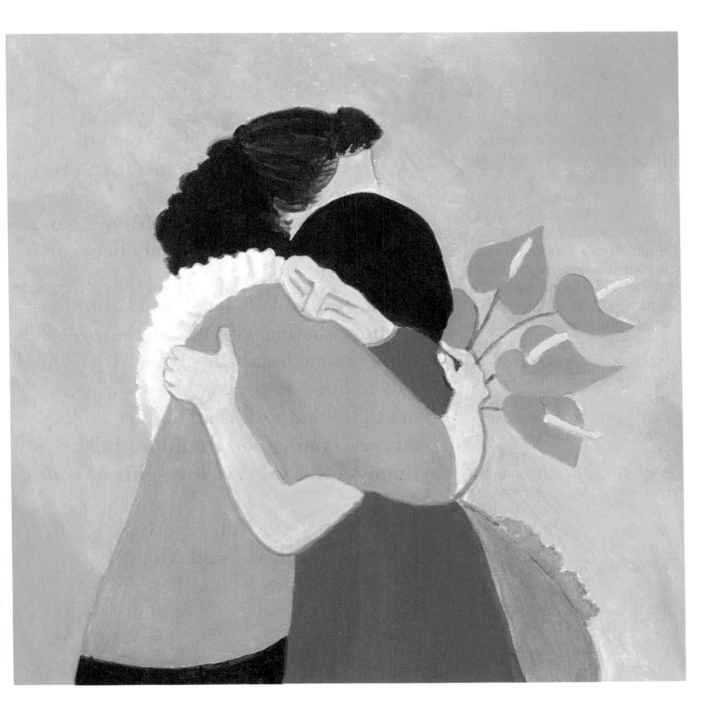

Parents wouldn't dream of poisoning their children. Yet many parents serve wrong foods daily without realizing their cumulative, damaging effects over time.

If one family member has diabetes, and everyone eats at the same family table, it's safe to assume those meals aren't promoting health. One person's illness can be the wake-up call that inspires healthy changes for the whole family. Family bonds can strengthen as everyone shares the challenge to change food choices and heal. When you become the role model, you make it easier for others to follow in your footsteps.

"*Passed* on, Mom," I corrected. "We're on a new track, remember? So let's make it stick."

I took Mili's hand and Mom's hand in mine and sandwiched them between my own. With pounding heart I said, "Mom, Aunty Mili, let's make a promise. No more sharing gifts of love that are really sickness time bombs in disguise. I want all of us to live healthy and long – I mean, isn't that what love is all about? So let's start *new* family food traditions full of yummy meals that are love-gifts of *health*. Deal?"

"Deal!" said Mili eagerly.

"Double-deal," said Mom.

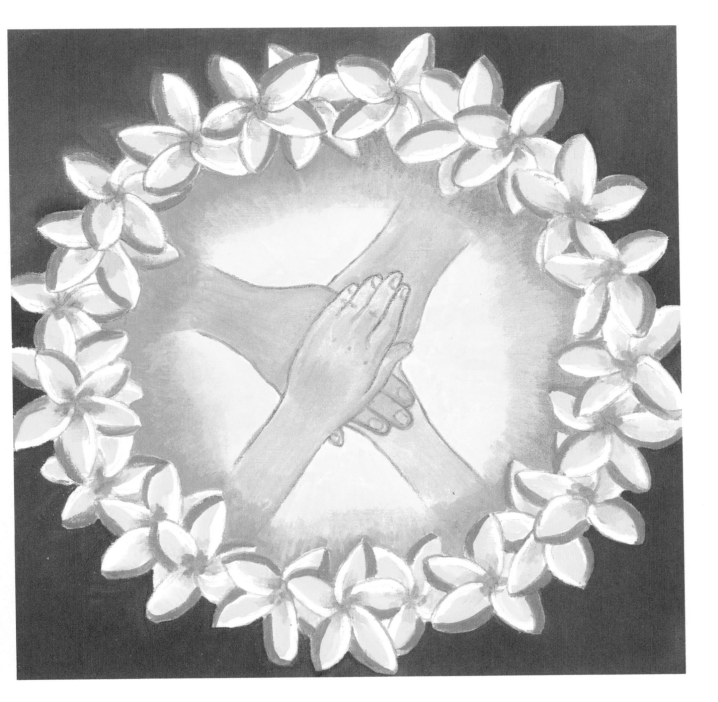

There's another medicine that benefits health. It's free. Nobody can give it to you or take it away from you. You get to choose it every day, and the choice is entirely up to you. What is it? It's your *attitude*. The way you feel and think about something affects how you act and what you achieve. A negative attitude helps keep you stuck and discouraged: *I can't. I don't want to. I know I won't like it.* A positive attitude helps you move forward: *I can. I'll try it. Maybe I'll like it.* Attitude spells the difference between ignoring knowledge and using that knowledge to change your life.

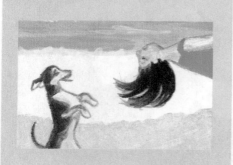

Aunty Mili was right. My taste buds changed. I could now taste the sweetness of real whole foods. And best of all, my food cravings vanished. One day I noticed that those sweet, fat, salty, processed foods had lost their power to grab me. That was huge!

Changing my food habits wasn't all easy. In fact, beating those addictive foods was downright hard. But I think that's the way most good things are. When you love yourself, you want to do good things for yourself. I want to feed my body what it needs to be strong. I want to give my mind what it needs to be focused. And I want to share my story with you, so you'll know that what I did *you can do too!*

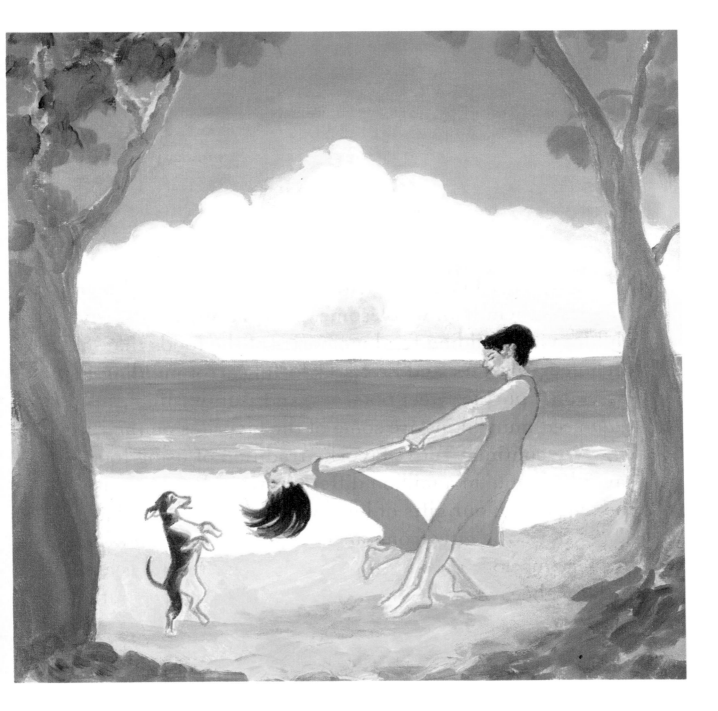

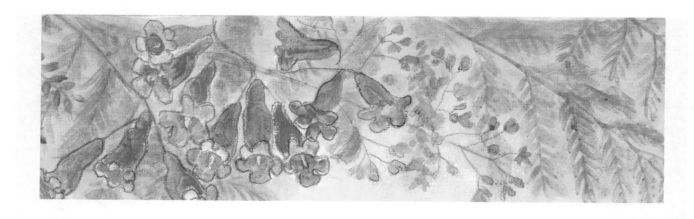

Now that I'm grown with two little boys of my own, I nourish them with wholesome, plant-happy meals. My children are building fond memories of the foods that make them feel cared for and loved. Colorful carrot pudding-cups, fat-bellied purple sweet potatoes, and Aunty Mili's *Mila*-seed munchkins are some of the favorites on their list.

We continue Tutu's favorite tradition of using food to say 'I love you' in a million different ways. But gone are the days when our gifts of love were toxic time bombs! These days, the gifts from our hearts carry love *and healing* in every luscious bite. My heart feels so grateful it soars with joy, because this, I know, *is* what love is all about.

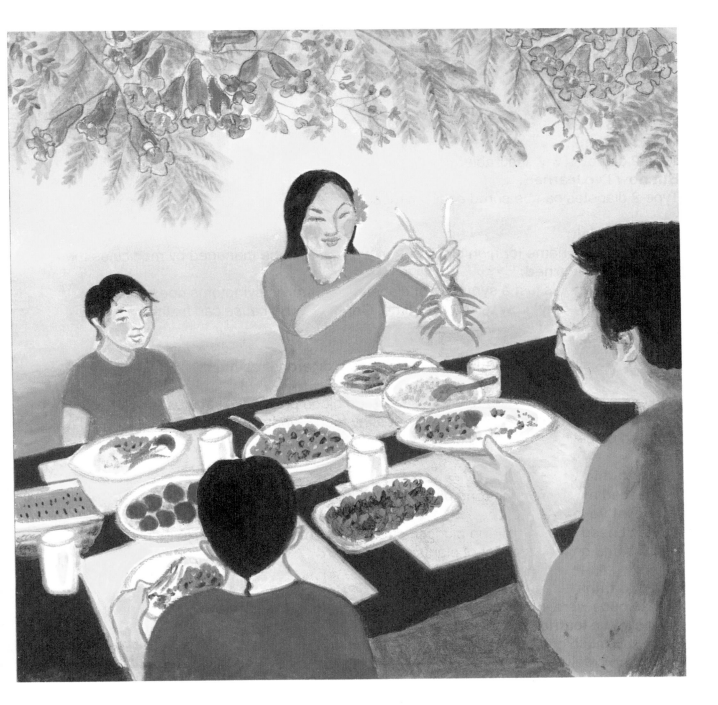

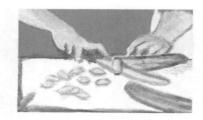

I used to think:
Type 2 diabetes was incurable.
But now I've learned:
Type 2 diabetes can be cured easily in most people.

I used to think:
Diabetes was a name for high blood sugar, which had to be managed by medicines for life.
But now I've learned:
High blood sugar is just a symptom of diabetes. Controling symptoms doesn't fix the problem, which may grow worse over time. Only fixing the *cause* can fix the problem.

I used to think:
Every disease has a different cause and needs a different treatment.
But now I've learned:
Lots of diseases – including heart disease, high blood pressure, diabetes, and many cancers – are fueled by eating unhealthy foods, and can be prevented and reversed by eating a balanced diet of whole plant foods.

I used to think:
We needed meat to build strong muscles and milk to build strong bones.
But now I've learned:
We don't need either one. The biggest, strongest animals on earth build their muscles and bones on a diet of plants.

I used to think:
Animal foods were important and necessary foods for building health.
But now I've learned:
Eating too much of these foods can make us fat and sick. We can get the nutrition we need more safely from a balanced diet of whole plant foods.

I used to think:
Eating sweets, sodas, and refined foods couldn't be so bad because 'everybody does it,'
and 'they wouldn't sell it to us if it really made us sick.'
But now I've learned:
People sell food products to make money, and sometimes those products are unhealthy and
addictive. They taste great and make us feel good, while damaging our bodies in sneaky ways
that we don't quickly feel or see.

I used to think:
The doctor always knows what's best for my health.
But now I've learned:
Doctors can only practice what they've learned. Most medical doctors (MDs) don't learn about
whole food, plant-based nutrition in medical school or at diabetes conferences, which focus
on how to manage diabetes using technologies.

I used to think:
I would feel hungry, unsatisfied, and weak from eating only plants.
But now I've learned:
Eating plants is delicious and satisfying. And I have *more* energy, not less.

My mom said she used to think:
Life wouldn't be worth living if she had to give up the foods she loved – but
because of *me* she was willing to try.
Now she says:
Taste buds *do* change! Eating healthy foods gives her body pleasure, and makes her life
more joyful than she ever dreamed. Life feels *more* worth living than before.

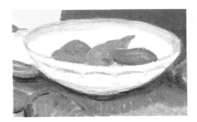

The following list is for those who want to learn more about the connection between food and health by exploring the books and DVDs in Aunty Mili's suitcase. The websites associated with many of these authors provide a wealth of free information including articles, newsletters, medical information, recipes, success stories, and support communities.

BOOKS:

The China Study, by T. Colin Campbell, PhD, and Thomas M. Campbell
http://www.thechinastudy.com and http://www.nutritionstudies.org

The End of Diabetes, by Joel Fuhrman, MD; http://www.drfuhrman.com

The Engine 2 Diet, by Rip Esselstyn; http://engine2diet.com

Forks Over Knives–The Cookbook, by Del Sroufe; http://www.forksoverknives.com

The Hawaii Diet Cookbook, by Terry Shintani, MD (book available at http://www.lulu.com)

Dr. Neal Barnard's Program for Reversing Diabetes, by Neal D. Barnard, MD
http://www.pcrm.org/health/ and http://www.nealbarnard.org

The Starch Solution, by John McDougall, MD, and Mary McDougall
http://www.drmcdougall.com

DVDs:

Dr Fuhrman's Secrets to Healthy Cooking
http://www.drfuhrman.com

Forks Over Knives; http://www.forksoverknives.com

Get Healthy Now DVD sets; http://www.vegsource.com

Latest in Clinical Nutrition DVDs; http://nutritionfacts.org

Simply Raw: Reversing Diabetes in 30 Days; http://www.rawfor30days.com

Tackling Diabetes with Dr. Neal Barnard; http://pcrm.org

Katherine Orr holds a certificate in plant-based nutrition from eCornell and the T. Colin Campbell Center for Nutrition Studies. To learn more about this program, visit http://www.nutritionstudies.org/.
To learn more about this and other books by Katherine, visit her website at http://www.KatherineShelleyOrr.com.

CPSIA information can be obtained at www.ICGtesting.com
Printed in the USA
BVOW10s2123110614

356154BV00001B/1/P